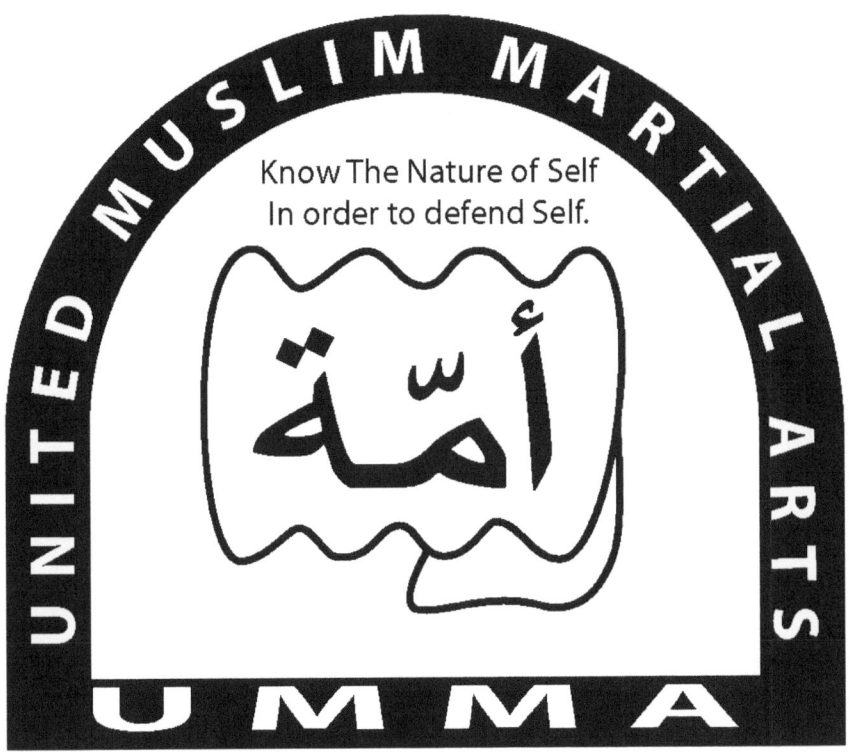

"Know The Nature Of Self, In Order To Defend Self"

- UMMA Chief Instructor Abdullah Sabree

www.ummamartialarts.com

Dedications

The authors dedicate this book to their loved ones. Our immediate families induce our greatest motivation. We will continue to make you proud.

Diaries Of A Mad Black Belt [Exercise Module] Revised Ed. is a work of non-fiction. Some names and identifying details have been altered.

Library of Congress cataloging-in-publication data

ISBN: 978-1-493-58025-5

Published in the United States of America

Diaries Of A Mad Black Belt

[Exercise Module]

Revised Ed.

Omar McKnight
Errol Seemangal

Table Of Contents

Prelude

Exercise Module

Supplementary Techniques

Afterword

Diaries Of A Mad Black Belt

[Exercise Module]

Revised Ed.

Omar McKnight
Errol Seemangal

[Prelude]

From Breakin' To Breakin'

After our Rap City interview and a slew of break-dance showcases, where we placed first in Canada's inaugural B-Boy Hip-Hop competition, we realized there would be a lot of people "hating". Still, we decided to celebrate anyway. Blitz and his boy Teeth chose to have an enjoyable night out at Latvian Hall on College St. in downtown Toronto. It was just the boys having harmless fun hanging out on the weekend….or so they thought.

One of the rival crews, The Tiny Tots, rolled up on Blitz mistaking him for someone else from a previous beef. The Tiny Tots were looking for revenge as a result of the preceding week's matter. As the crew zeroed in on Blitz, his natural aggressiveness did not immediately kick-in. Rather, he tried talking his way out of the situation. After indulging in the usual Friday night intoxicants, the setting for negotiations wasn't an option for the Tiny Tots.

Bam! Something hit Blitz from behind. Bang! Blitz momentarily thought he was watching a retro Batman episode with all the written sound effects. A nearby lady screamed "*AHHHH!*" while witnessing the assault. After being swarmed with kicks and punches for about twenty seconds, Blitz was down and out for the count. An adjacent light then quickly turned on and the assailants scattered like roaches.

Blitz thought the cowards should come show their faces and fight. Although, he was happy he wasn't seriously injured. A security guard asked if he was okay and he nodded yes. Teeth then finally caught up with Blitz but for some reason, the crew didn't target him. Was he the lucky one? Or, was it his destiny?

Both friends were thankful they made it out alive and recalled the proverb *"You can live like a mouse or die like a lion"*. To this day, both Blitz and Teeth still think about this old saying.

At The Crossroads

"Yo Blitz, I heard what happened. Man, are you okay?" a friend asked. He shook his head but wasn't in the mood for many words. On the inside, he realized he was dying slowly.

"We gotta get revenge now bro. How could you let this happen? We told you guys not to go out after the showcase. You knew there would be a lot of haters out there."

"Yeah, that's true" Blitz muttered.

"Just say the word and we get them!"

Blitz thought long and hard about revenge-murder but the longer he thought about it, the more he realized it wasn't worth it. He reflected on what path he was going to go down and how far he had come already. After his boy Kwame came by and they talked about what happened, Kwame said "Maybe this is your calling."

"Calling?" Blitz stated. He then deliberated further. He knew God was trying to tell him something. He also knew God worked in mysterious ways. Maybe he was being told that if he were to continue down this road his fate was either jail, serious injury, or …death!

"You should come to church this week man" Kwame assured.

For real Blitz thought. It was a good idea and he hadn't been in ages. Up until then, it was as though Hip-Hop was his only way of life.

The Awakening

Blitz went upstairs after his conversation, dusted off his *Qur'an*, made *wudu*, and began to pray. Later, he hooked up with some active Muslim brothers and joined a self-defense class. He reasoned it would be productive to learn some life skills and street knowledge too. Enhancing his spirituality would be another benefit he figured.   He felt it wasn't necessary "to fit in" to be respected. Blitz also remembered a verse of the *Qur'an* he once read. It was a powerful statement that remained embedded in his head.

Is it honor, power, and glory that they seek? Well to Allah belongs all the honor, power, and glory. . ." (35:10)

It has been seventeen years since this all happened. From breakin' on stage in front of thousands to martial-arts breakin' and spiritual awakening. Maybe Blitz's past of ignorance had facilitated this new transcendence. No matter how things change, they remain the same.

The *Qur'an* is the scared Islamic text

wudu means to perform the ablution

Karmic Debt

When thinking back to all those years of neglecting spirituality, the authors realize this is where real contentment and fulfillment lie. Moreover, we feel obligated to give back to our past and present communities. In doing so, we hope to steer those following a similar negative path into a 180 degree turn. We will try our best to be role models by helping people regardless of gender, color, race, age, or background.

Some may say "Guidance! Guidance!". When you are given a second chance in life, you do everything as if it's your last opportunity. We can never really do enough because we're eternally in debt to *Allah*. With every breath, we are given an additional occasion to be shining examples.

Allah is an Arabic word meaning (the one) God

The "Blessed" Seed

In herbal medicine, nigella sativa has hypertensive, carminative, and anthelminthic properties according to various sources. It has been traditionally used for a variety of conditions and treatments related to respiratory health, stomach and intestinal health, kidney and liver function, circulatory and immune system support, and for general well-being.

A well known *hadith* relating to this seed follows:

According to Abu Hurairah, he says, "I heard Allah's Apostle saying, 'There is healing in black cumin for all diseases except death.'" [1]

Black seed has been heralded as the blessed seed. Personally, I have found the benefits of black seed to be simply amazing. As a baby, ever since I could remember, I suffered from bronchitis. So, whenever winter came I would succumb to nasty colds and had to seek antibiotics... or so I thought. But now using this herb, I rarely get sick. If I do, my immune system recovers very well. Black seed is truly an immune system enhancer.

For martial-arts, black seed increases my stamina while exercising. I can truly say it is a blessed herb. I recommend taking it as prescribed, but I use it in capsule form twice a day after a big meal. Then you are ready to say *"Hieeee-Yaaaaah!"*

A *hadith* is a saying, teaching, or practice of the prophet Muhammad (peace be upon him)

[1] *Sahih Bukhari* 7. 592

Introduction

The following exercise module consists of short log chronicles. They consist of my experiences in the dojo. Its purpose is to encourage people to live a healthy lifestyle physically, mentally, and spiritually. It is through martial-arts one can learn teamwork, their strengths and weaknesses, and how to overcome obstacles they may face. Martial-arts can also serve as a safeguard from bad elements. We hope our efforts are beneficial and fun for those who wish to perform any of the exercises outlined. Lastly, we have included YouTube links of the exercises for those who are visual learners.

[Exercise Module]

Grade "A" Material

With Chief Instructor Abdullah Sabree
09/16/06
Etobicoke, Ontario, Canada
United Muslim Martial Arts (UMMA) Headquarters

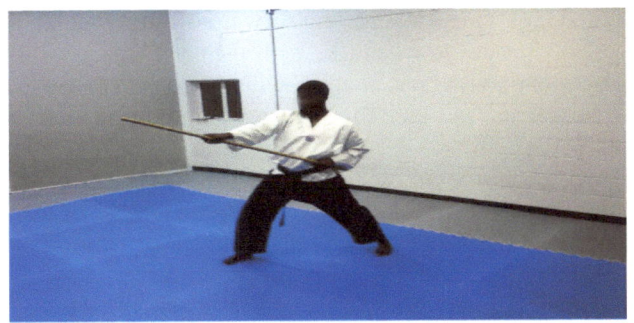

http://youtu.be/ooEEbhM5POo

Surprise Grading Anyone?

Yes, even black belts must get graded. However, to make things interesting it was a surprise bo-staff grading. Yikes! To be exact, it was more of an unofficial grading, similar to an in-class pop quiz. Nonetheless, it was a grading.

Shishnee-kun, the first tournament pattern, was what we were tested on. At first, I froze at the beginning and had a lot of mistakes but managed to wobble my way through. I scored a measly 5/10. My second time around I did a little better scoring 7/10. I think the bad gripping and lack of practice plagued me each time.

This day was quite embarrassing and uplifting all in one. We had a grading for the color belts which was always fun because we found out who had been "naughty or nice" with their techniques.

We then had our black belt class in which we worked on combinations of kicking, punching, and endurance. Listed are the sequences we completed:

- double side-kick moving forward off the front leg
- reverse hook-kick off the back leg
- reverse roundhouse kick stepping with the in-step of the foot first
- jab, punch, axe-kick (off the back leg), reverse kick [2]

Finally as black belts do, we brought it back to the basics of patterns. We always for go over each pattern. Repetition is the mother of learners a wise man once said.

The class main benefit here was the fact I got to see where I was in terms of the bo-staff. I was reminded that anything can happen at any given time, even in the dojo. Well, it was better to have happened in practice than in a real life situation for sure.

---

[2] This combination works well due of the fluidity of the techniques and is meant to flow like water

Memory Lane

04/15/08
Etobicoke, Ontario, Canada
United Muslim Martial Arts (UMMA) Headquarters

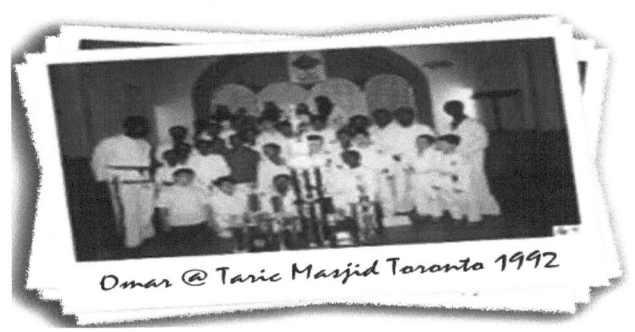

Omar @ Taric Masjid Toronto 1992

Sometimes, life may get in the way even when you have a passion for something. People can change but their drive maybe rekindled and you find yourself back on the ones and twos.

This class was a walk down memory lane because my fellow colleague, Nabil Hack, joined us from Taric Martial Arts. The chronological order of this particular class follows. Feel free to follow along.

1. Warm-Up

- jogging around the dojo, stop, ten push-ups then switch directions

- from sitting stance, 3 punches (low, medium, high) (10 repetitions)

- leg stretching and leg raises (10 repetitions)

- worm push-ups to the wall and back

- side-kick with both legs (10 repetitions)

- front-snap kick 10 with both legs (repetitions)

- push-ups, run to the wall and back
- crouch hopping with your hands on your head to the wall and back

Then there was an explanation of how your supporting foot supports the round-house kick.

- then we did round-house kicks (10 repetitions)

Chief Instructor Abdullah Sabree then stepped in to continue class

2. Combinations

- lounge punch with each hand (20 repetitions)

- reverse punch with each hand (20 repetitions)

- front-snap kick with each leg (20 repetitions)

- then we combined all techniques and added a *kiai*

After combinations, we practiced our patterns. We had to help Nabil since it had been so long for him. The upside of teaching someone patterns is you actually reinforce the movements for yourself. Finally, everyone sparred but I mainly helped out with the lower belts.

The takeaway of this class was helping others and remembering to follow instructions. Just because you don't see someone for a while you should take the initiative to find out how they are doing. Assisting others by sacrificing your time and effort can be rewarding if done for the right reasons.

Hip-Hapkido!

With Dr. Hassan Al-Misree
01/04/09
Scarborough, Ontario, Canada
Islamic Foundation of Toronto

Having Dr. Hassan lead the class was a special treat because he studied Karate and Hapkido in Japan. The class was also attended by Errol Seemangal, one of my longtime students. Dr. Hassan outlined sparring techniques that I think are the foundation of any fight. Below are descriptions of the exercises he taught.

Sen-sen
Sen-sen is all about anticipation. Once your attacker initiates an advance, you advance too but jimmy off to one side. You then inner-forearm block any strike aimed at your body. Next, you counter with a reverse punch. Or, use the palm of your hand if you're not wearing gloves. I noticed with sen-sen, that clashes are common and you may get slightly injured. But, you've got to take a little to give a little sometimes. Although, the more you practice the better off you will be.

Atono-sen
Atono-sen is about feinting. Essentially, you open-up your attacker by faking a move such as throwing your hands up and then front-snap kicking or check-kicking low. Your attacker may attempt to block low. If so, you then throw a head-level kick instead seeking a knockout.

Gono-sen
With this technique, you dodge an attacker's move and counter-attack. Or, perform a self defense takedown move such as an arm lock and punch. If attacked with a round-house kick, take the hit. This will open-up your attacker and leave them vulnerable. Then, counter with a reverse hook-kick or similar strike.

The lesson from this class was to do what works best for you.   Knowing your true nature is the best defense. Another point was to keep familiar with like minded martial artists as to stay fluid at all times.

Reflexes, Self Defense, And Patterns

With Head Instructor Abu Yazdan
04/09/10
Hamilton, Ontario, Canada
Muslim Community of Hamilton

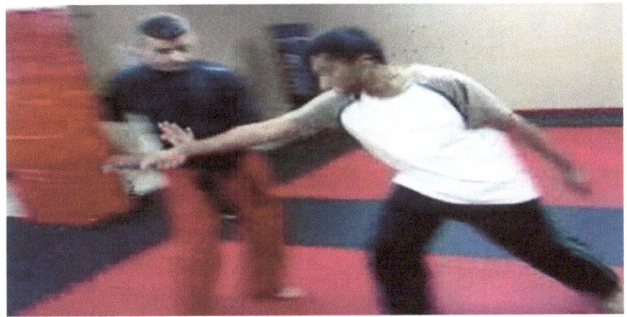

Head Instructor Abu Yazdan and Harris
Knife defense techniques

http://youtu.be/HPocE6qviYk

To begin, we practiced some reflex exercises including a block-secure-punch technique which is detailed below.

Both you and a partner face each other in ready-stance. One partner steps with their right foot while simultaneously punching with their right hand. The other partner steps diagonally with the right foot, weaves, and open hand blocks with their left hand. The defender then secures the attacker's wrist with their left hand and counters with a right punch.

After practicing the technique several times, we switched to defending a left punch. Attacker and defender roles were reversed and we continued to execute the exercise.

Bear Hug Or Full Nelson Self Defense

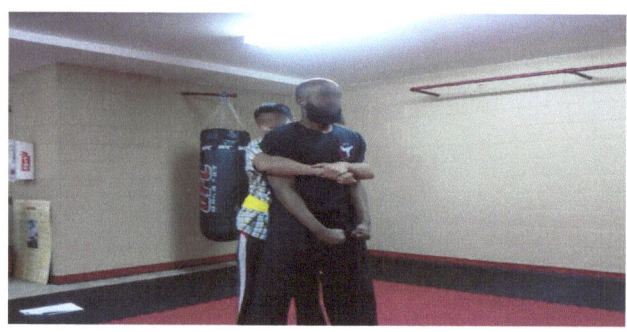

http://youtu.be/3RAXrAkoVew

The attacker starts off by bear-hugging the defender from behind. Next, the defender uses either of their legs to step to the opposite side of attacker and spin. The attacker and defender should now be face to face. After that, the defender uses their arms to break free or can drop-slide to the floor and head for safety.

Patterns

International Taekwondo Federation (ITF) 5th Pattern

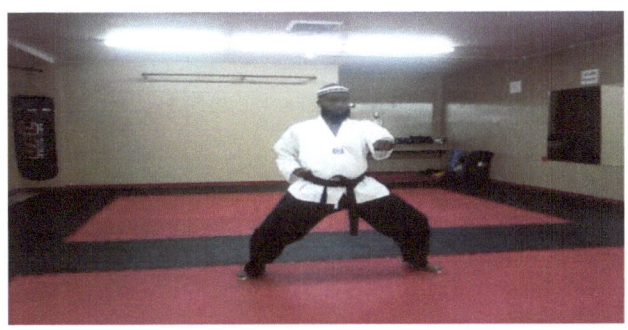

http://youtu.be/Luunw-h9x3E

The fifth pattern is a transitional pattern that focuses on breathing regulation and strengthening your abdominal muscles. It's a great pattern to warm-up to when participating in tournaments. Moreover it's a great workout, if done correctly, all by itself.

In this class I learned another technique to utilize in close range. I was able to get a sense of what to do when in close quarters with an attacker. It was also nice to improve my reflexive skills and timing.

Patterns As A Warm-up?

07/10/10
Hamilton, Ontario, Canada
Muslim Community of Hamilton

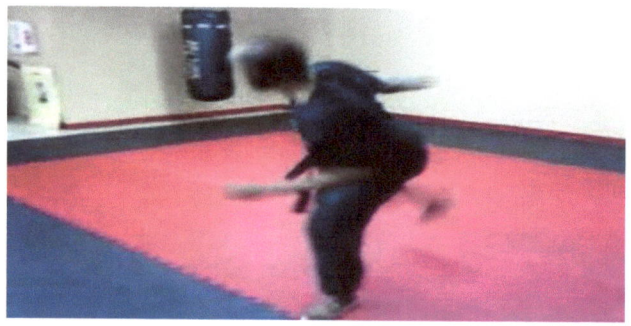

http://youtu.be/owrt7gK27wA

We started off performing patterns as our warm-up. Sometimes, just executing patterns repeatedly can get boring. Instead, we broke the patterns down into each particular movement. This was phenomenal because we rehearsed each movement several times. For example every punch, kick, or block was done ten times each. Needless to say, this made for a great warm-up. This method ensured you focused on correct form.

Next, we moved onto kicking techniques. From a fighting-stance, we did forty front-snap kicks off the front leg then forty off the back leg. After that, we would take a step with our back leg and front-snap kick off the front leg. We also did this forty times with each leg.

Later we each got a chair and performed as many step-ups and decline pushups as we could. Subsequently, we did crab walks and army crawls back and forth across the dojo.

We finished off with Hapkido self defense techniques including the locking of the wrists and arms. With a partner, we would take turns carrying out wrist takedowns continuously. We also practiced thumb pressure-point takedowns.

The moral from this class was the pattern repetition. Mastery of any technique requires repeated practice using the right form. After all, they say repetition is the mother of learners.

The Warm-Up

With Sensei Khalil
01/03/11
Hamilton, Ontario, Canada
Muslim Community of Hamilton

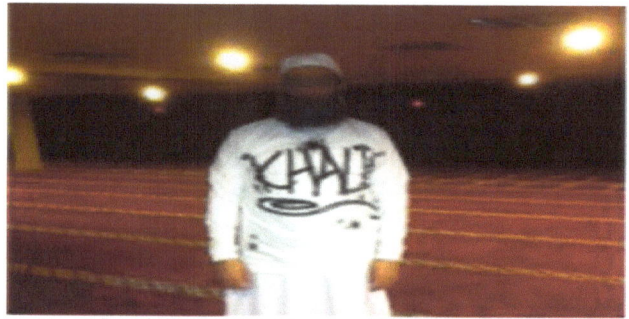

Sensei Khalil has over ten years teaching experience

Sensei Khalil had us run around the dojo to warm-up. After a few laps, we began to punch with every step for another few laps. I found this a very good warm-up because running doesn't involve the upper body much. But, running and punching combined makes it much more exciting.

The class continued onto self-defense exercises. For example, an attacker would grab the defender from behind and over the defender's arms. The defender would then stun the attacker using any strike, such as an elbow and then hip toss them using either leg.

Our warm-down included jogging in one spot and we eventually turned it into a game. When Sensei Khalil clapped once, we did two push-ups. When he clapped twice, we did two sit-ups followed by jogging and kicking up our heels as fast as we could for one minute. We concluded with backwards break-falls on both sides and tried to get up without using the hands.

This class was very beneficial because it was executed as realistic as possible. When the attacker grabs, it is as though it would happen on the street. You are forced to react in a practical manner to see if the techniques would work for you.

Friday Night Madness

Omar vs. Fahad Qureshi
01/10/11
Hamilton, Ontario, Canada
Muslim Community of Hamilton

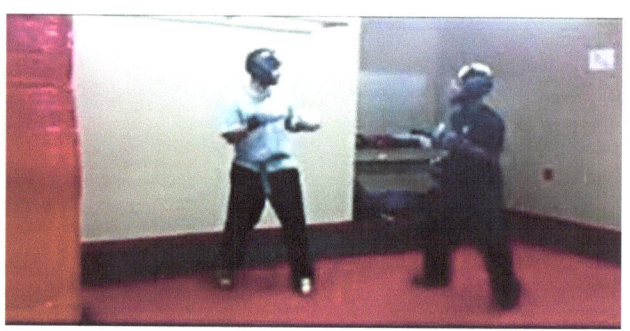

http://youtu.be/gaz0jWYS3RM

The title of this entry was inspired by the fact that Friday is when people usually get wild and crazy. However, we do so in a calm martial arts manner by letting our skills speak. And, without the hangovers. Ha!

We started warming up with one-hundred jumping jacks and punching ten times each with both hands back and forth. We then moved onto ten knee-ups with each leg followed by ten front- snap kicks with each leg. After adding a double punch to the front-snap kicks we did some stretching, and took a break for *salah*.

After returning, we started to spar. I was coaching the students and telling the colored belts which combinations work best for their individual fighting style. I also reminded them to *kiai* on their knockout strikes. After a while of watching, I got tired of telling people what to do. It was time to lead by example! So, I suited up my sparring gear and got in the ring.

I sparred the lower belts to get warmed up. Surprisingly, I got hit in the eye because I didn't block properly. Ouch! Yusuf, a brother who practices jiu-jitsu, had some really good boxing combinations. He did, however, over-praise me. Later, I finally got in the groove and scored good combinations myself using my *kiai* techniques. Another brother, Mohammed, ended the match and mentioned I should incorporate reverse punch into my repertoire.

This class reiterated the fact that I shouldn't be teaching all the time. I should be an active participant to keep my skills sharp. As a teacher, partaking with the students sometimes makes the class more interesting overall.

Salah means prayer and is the second pillar of Islam

Kiai is a short vocalization used during a technique

ObScUre Obstacles

02/05/11
Hamilton, Ontario, Canada
Muslim Community of Hamilton

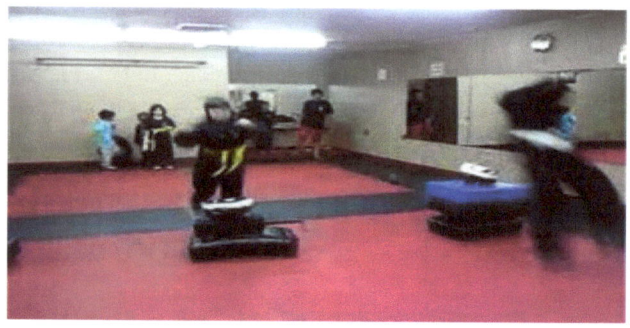

http://youtu.be/Gj7hmm9IU4k

This class was quite obscure to say the least! We started off with about ten laps around the dojo and one lap of crouch hopping. We raised our knees up while jogging and took big swing steps. As laps continued, two students would perform five chin-ups on the bars on the wall and then continue jogging. The students switched and did a total of three sets.

After that, we slowed down a bit. Mohammed put up huge square punching pads in the middle of the dojo and we started jumping over them with two-footed vertical jumps. We ensured our knees were tucked-in and executed the technique one by one.

After everyone completed three jumps Mohammed would increase the height using anything he could find. It was reminiscent of a high-jump track meet. If you didn't clear a specific height, you had to do ten push-ups. It was an extraordinary exercise, but fun. After taking a break, we partnered up and did three sets of twenty push-ups and thirty crunches.

Punching Bag Practice
Once the bag was setup, we took turns kicking with twenty front-snap kicks, twenty side-kicks, twenty round-house kicks, and twenty crescent-kicks. It was a bit tiring but gave us a chance to work on the power of our kicks.

We finished off by socializing about random topics. The lower belts admired my crescent-kicks for which I gladly said thanks. The students asked the teacher about advanced kicking techniques, but he reminded them to just stick to the basics.

I mentioned that being a black belt meant mastering your basic techniques. Fancy styles are mainly for demonstration purposes. I also stated that on the street it doesn't take much to overpower aggressors.

Hygiene, Hygiene, Hygiene!

(Jiu-Jitsu Class)
03/20/11
Hamilton, Ontario, Canada
Muslim Community of Hamilton

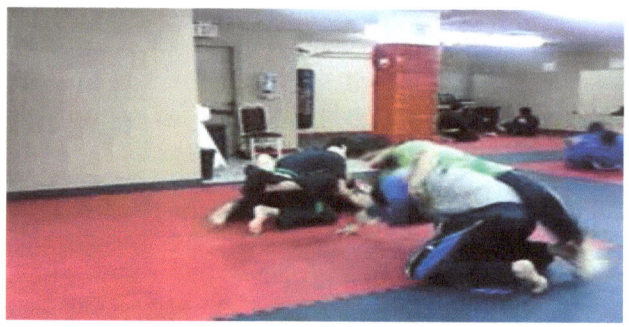

http://youtu.be/kS0UdNFS1EA

Sensei Yusuf was back in town from a work-related trip and it was nice to have him back. On occasion, life can get in the way of martial arts. But, you can never keep a good man down.

He started off by reminding us to have proper attire especially when practicing jiu-jitsu. Many people have caught bad diseases because they lacked adequate dress.

After that we started our warm-ups: jogging around the dojo in single file for ten laps, sideways shuffling for ten laps, and weaving our legs sideways for ten laps. We then jogged with our knees up and jogged by kicking our heels back into our backsides (talk about a self-inflicted wound). Next, we touched the wall then sprinted to the opposite wall and slowed down by walking.

Subsequent to that, came bear-walking. This exercise requires you to get on all fours and walk as if you were a four-legged animal similar to a caveman. This is a particularly great workout when done continuously. It forces you to focus on your core muscle groups and balance.

We moved onto the next exercise which consisted of one person in front of the line stopping and turning 15 degrees in push-up position. The rest of the line army-crawled under him to form a worm. The last person had to crawl under the entire line and start all over again for one lap. We then lined up by twos and each person did break falls in single file backwards while rolling out of it.

Then came sparring time jiu-jitsu style! The instructor told us to spar at 30% for ten minutes. It had been a while since I was back in class, so it was a great workout. I got the opportunity to burn some extra calories off my chest…or should I say waist?

As the class continued, we worked on the following sitting headlock technique: from behind your partner, grab and place them into a headlock making sure your elbow is facing the same direction as them. With your other hand, grab your opposite bicep (one of your hands should be holding the back of your partner's head tilting it forward). You then flex your muscles and squeeze moving both arms in the direction of the partner's head. If done correctly, this technique results in an automatic submission or tap-out as it's really painful!

The Sensei reiterated the importance of hygiene and things to be mindful of when practicing jiu-jitsu. Specifically, skin diseases are common because of close contact and exchange of sweat during matches. What you should do is take a shower before and after every session, regularly cut the finger and toenails, and wear a t-shirt or rash guard under your uniform. A spandex t-shirt may help as well.

Just Kids Part I

10/19/12
Hamilton, Ontario, Canada
Muslim Community of Hamilton

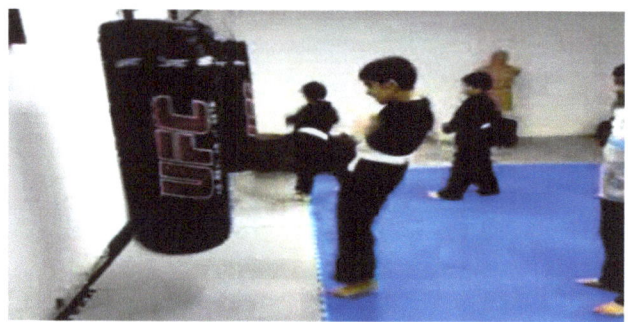

Today was my first day teaching on a Monday, so I wasn't used to it. Everything that could have delayed me did. First, I forgot my keys. Then, I received calls from my parents. After that, I realized I didn't have my belt with me. But, with every difficulty there comes ease. I told my parents I was running late so I could run around to the back side of the dojo to open the doors. I miraculously found a spare black belt in a nearby closet and quickly tied it on. I guess things always seem to work out for the best with good intention and effort. So, the fun began.

    1. Warm-Up

- jogging on the spot, ten laps (five push-ups, five sit-ups every second lap), stretching, ten leg raises with each leg, and crouch-hopping back and forth across the dojo

2. Kicking Review:

We first reviewed the basics of the front-snap kick by number

     i.   Raise the knee (i.e. "chamber" the knee)

    ii.   Extend the leg while simultaneously bending the toes backwards

   iii.   Retract the leg back into chambering position

   iv.   Return the leg into fighting-stance

Then we performed the kick ten times at full speed with each leg. After that, we performed the technique moving across the entirety of the dojo.

We also reviewed the basics of the side-kick by number

     i.   Chamber the knee

    ii.   Pivot the supporting foot 90 degrees and extend the kicking leg

            (while turning your body to the side)

   iii.   Retract the leg back into chambering position

   iv.   Return the leg into fighting-stance

Instead of executing the kick with no target, I got the heavy bag and told the kids to line up. This way, they would experience the realism of each kick.

The kids' attention span is very short so I had to keep things interesting. Thus, we finished off with a game of chicken which seemed to help with their balance, stability, and competitiveness. Their will to succeed also seemed to shine through.

My takeaway from this class was remembering what is important. What's significant is the act of training itself. Proper dress is vital too, but to a lesser extent. I also remembered to adjust the class to the students' skill level no matter how advanced or experienced they were.

Just (Big) Kids Part II

04/06/13
Hamilton, Ontario, Canada
Muslim Community of Hamilton

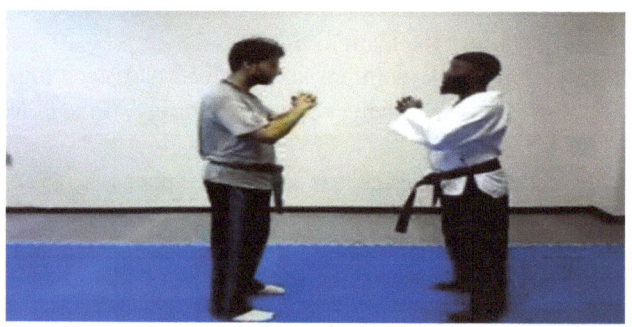

This day the class was full of adults who varied in age. Adults always seem to be more ready and eager than kids. So, there was little talk and we got right to action.

The class started off with twenty laps with ten push-ups and sit-ups every other lap. We quickly did full body stretching and then proceeded to sitting-stance combinations.

The first combination executed was five sets of three punches to the high, medium, and low positions. The second was ten sets of two front-snap kicks per count for a total of twenty kicks. Other combinations practiced were side-kick, back-fist, reverse punch and front snap-kick, low-section block, reverse punch, then back-kick.

After practicing Hapkido wrist-grab exercises, we did some boxing conditioning for fifteen second intervals for twenty minutes. The students seemed tired at this point so we proceeded to bo-staff practice for green belts and higher.

The bo-staff itself is similar to four weapons combined into one. It is the combination of staff, sword, stick, and nun-chucks. It is also an extension of the hand so a lot of moves mimic basic hand techniques such as turning the wrist over during striking and blocking.

The students had come a long way and were ecstatic to weapons train. To warm-up, we did figure-eights which looked as if the students had improved on since the last time. I fine tuned their strikes and blocks for reiteration purposes.

Time was running so we practiced the first pattern shish-nee-kun first by number and then on timing. I noticed their memory of the pattern still existed but subtle details were sometimes omitted. I reminded them to practice at home with a broom-stick or other similar object. If no object was available I still told them to rehearse the movements so it would become second nature.

The message of this class was that age shouldn't be a hindrance. This principle isn't restricted to martial arts. Goals should be pursued regardless of age. It isn't too late to get fit. It isn't too late to seek further education. It isn't too late to make a difference. It isn't too late to achieve your objectives.

[Supplementary Techniques]

Block To Basics:

(1a) High Section Block

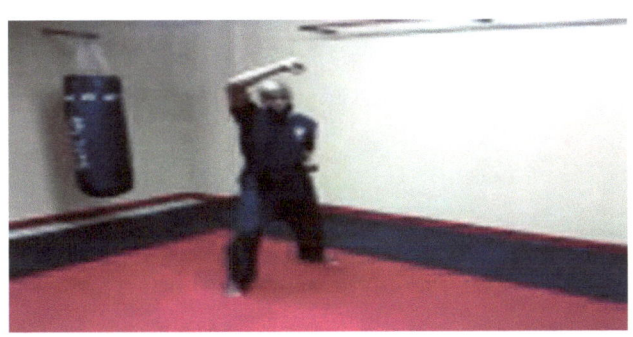

http://youtu.be/cfM5yriqx58

High section block is one of the most common and effective blocks in martial arts. Ideally, you want to make sure the forearm is 45 degrees above head-level. And, of course, you turn your wrist over at the last second as if you were striking. So if an attack were to come from above, it merely slides off the arm. You could then counterattack and head to safety. Enjoy and have fun! Be safe.

(1b)   Low Section Block

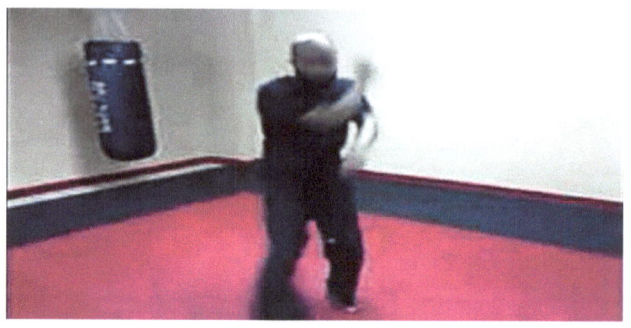

http://youtu.be/a03SyRYMj6k

Another great way to stay safe and protect the body from harm is the low section block. If an attack is coming from the waist or below, you want to make sure to execute this technique. And again, for emphasis, turning the wrist over is crucial to making the block work. When the block is performed, your hand should be just above the knee cap (when in a walking-stance position). Another secret I want to share is turning your hips over provides more power and stability as you may see in the video demonstration. Do not try to be a hero.

(1c)   Inner-Forearm Block

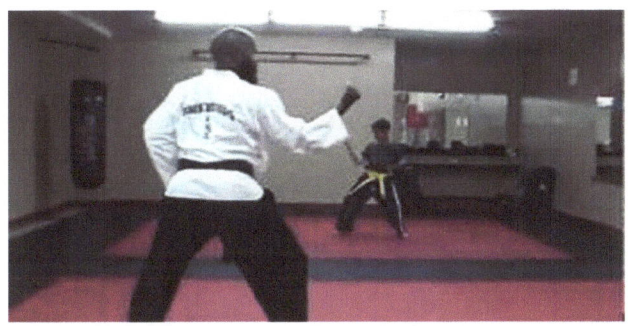

http://youtu.be/tiYixEGTfEs

In this section we focus on the inner-forearm block. Generally speaking, this block defends the chest area of the body. It is important to note that turning the wrist over, like the aforementioned blocks, is essential to proper execution.   One benefit of blocking the mid-section of the body is that recovering to counterattack becomes easier. Counters originating from this position take less time than other block positions.   For example, a quick jab or back-hand may back your aggressor away.

(2) Forearm Strengthening

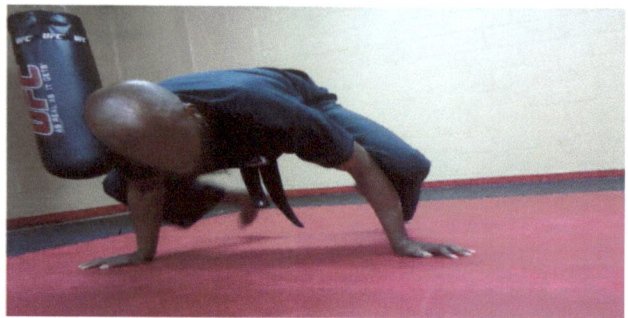

An alternative forearm strengthening exercise

http://youtu.be/GXvLZ8TYflk

Having strong forearms is essential for the three previously mentioned blocks. It is the forearms that usually absorb strikes and protect the body. Thus fortifying this part of the body is pivotal.

This is a three-part exercise that works the wrists and forearm muscles. First, each partner performs a wind-up block swinging their right hand into their partner's right hand. The same block is then performed with the left hand. Second, an outside-inside block is then carried out with the right hand and stops at your partner's right hand. The same block is then performed with the left hand. Third, a low section block is then performed with the right hand which stops at the partner's right hand. The same block is then performed with the left hand completing six total blocks.

(3) A-Bowl-A-Punch!

(Reverse Punch)

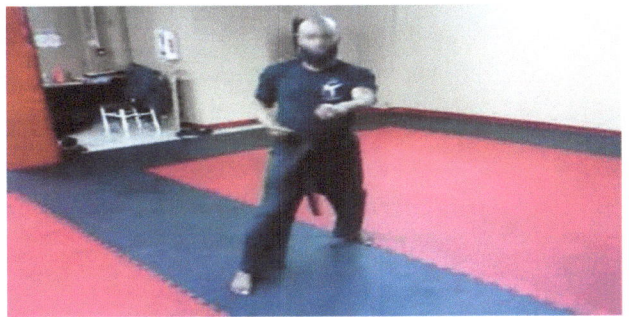

http://youtu.be/RnWat1TZkig

This is a brief lesson on the foundations of punching. Specifically, reverse punch, which involves a step with either leg and a punch with the opposite arm. Using the hips and turning your wrist over is essential too. The key aspect about martial arts techniques is to work smarter, not harder. Applying the proper execution and timing will exert less energy, which are vital when it comes to sustaining endurance.

(4) Bobbing and Weaving

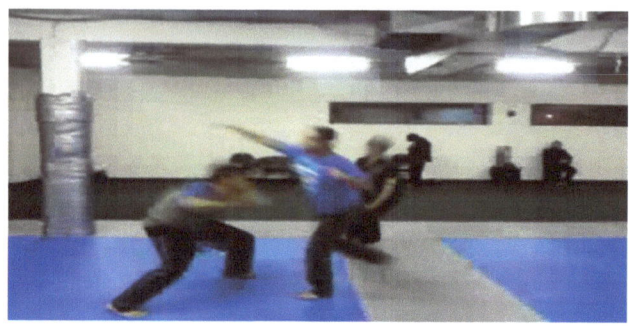

http://www.youtube.com/watch?feature=player_embedded&v=etm2sPd2w9Y

Proper defensive prowess is imperative to staying out of harm's way. Moving with correct form can literally mean the difference between life and death. Bobbing and weaving are staple moves of a fighter in order to avoid being struck in close contact situations. Practical applications of this technique could come in handy when foiling a robbery attempt. At times, a front-snap kick may not be the best option so bobbing or weaving then counter-attacking could deter aggressors.

(5)   Balance

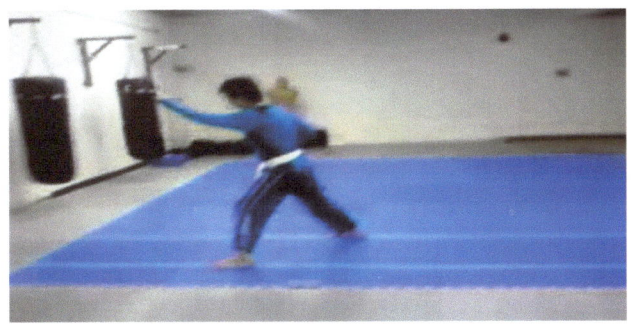

http://www.youtube.com/watch?feature=player_embedded&v=tQMycphYtIw

Balance is not just essential for martial arts, but it's crucial in everyday life too. One factor in maintaining proper balance is the abdominal muscles. Contracting the core muscles, including those of the lower back and back-side, play roles in maintaining good posture.

Another aspect of balance deals with being ambidextrous. If you're right-handed, it is important to develop your left limbs to be as effective and agile as your right limbs. Practicing patterns is one way to advance your non-dominant side. Remember, anything can happen at any time so disregarding consequences could be fatal.

(6)   The Bo-Staff

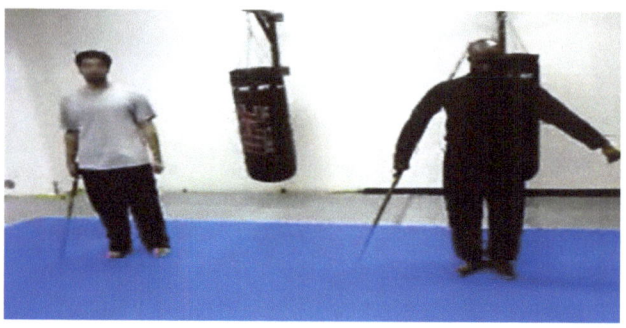

http://www.youtube.com/watch?feature=player_embedded&v=1084jXFMTBs

The bo-staff is a cardiovascular workout all by itself. It accelerates the heart rate and works the arm muscles simultaneously.   However, weapons shouldn't be taught to students who have not obtained, at least, the green belt.

One thing to keep in mind with the bo-staff is the push-pull theory. For instance, when attempting a cross-strike one end of the staff (a push) the other end should be drawn towards your body (a pull) with equal force.

[Afterword]

Author Biographies

Omar McKnight

Omar was born in 1975 in Toronto, Ontario, Canada. His parents had earlier emigrated from the Caribbean. At the age of 19, Omar had a near death experience involving gangs. This event initiated his accepting Islam. In 1995, Omar joined United Muslim Martial Arts (UMMA) which was formerly Taric Martial Arts. He studied Taekwondo under the guide of Chief Instructor Abdullah Sabree and became a black belt in 2000. This was followed by a brown belt in bo-jitsu from Patrice Belle.

Omar has taught, competed, and demonstrated martial arts at various events across Ontario. He currently lives with his family in Hamilton where he teaches at the Mountain *Masjid* and studies jiu-jitsu. Omar also enjoys graphic design and marketing. To learn more about Omar, visit his website www.omarmcknight.com.

Errol Seemangal

Errol was also born and raised in Toronto but currently resides in the United States. He started training under Omar and the UMMA organization in 2005. In the summer of 2009, Errol relocated to Baltimore, Maryland, U.S.A and continued training with AAA U.S. Taekwondo College. He subsequently received his black belt in 2013.

Errol hopes to one day extend the UMMA brand into the U.S. to capitalize on the popularity of martial arts. His other aspirations include pursuing a doctorate degree and publishing additional books. His interests include sports, fitness, music, and traveling. To learn more about Errol, visit his website www.errolseemangal.com.

Masjid is a synonym for mosque

Acknowledgments

The authors would like to recognize those who played central roles in the inspiration of this book. Above all, all praise are due to Allah (*swt*). Nothing is possible without Him. Moreover, gratitude is sent to His last messenger (peace be upon him). We are grateful to be continuously shown the straight path. *Ameen.*

Next, we must give thanks to all our instructors. Principally, we highlight Chief Instructor Abdullah Sabree of the UMMA. We also show appreciation to Master Instructors Paul Lewis and Tim Beach of AAA U.S. Taekwondo College.

Mcknight Thank Yous

I must thank Toronto West Side, Complex, Woolner Avenue, Bag of Trix, Granny, T&T, Denise, Jamal, Tahanee, Khaleelah, and Claudette. Also, appreciation goes out to Runnyemede Collegiate, Suliman,Taric Masjid, Troid, Hamilton Masjid, and Abu Shahadah. I'd also like to give a special thanks to my wife and the Shaikh family. I would not be in the position I am in now without them.

Seemangal Thank Yous

I'd like to thank my parents. Decades ago, it was them who decided to move to the West for better opportunity. Thus, I was the recipient of great educational and business opportunities. For that, I must thank them.

swt is an abbreviation for *subḥānahu wa ta'āla*. Its translation is "May He be Glorified and Exalted"

Notes

Notes